Distribution, publication, and copying in any form are prohibited and subject to damages.

TEN HYPNOSES

Copying, publishing, and sharing with third parties are only permitted with the written consent of the author. Please observe the notes on copyright and usage.

Distribution, publication, and copying in any form are prohibited and subject to damages.

Copying, publishing, and sharing with third parties are only permitted with the written consent of the author. Please observe the notes on copyright and usage.

Distribution, publication, and copying in any form are prohibited and subject to damages.

Ingo Michael Simon

TEN HYPNOSES

3

BURNOUT

Copying, publishing, and sharing with third parties are only permitted with the written consent of the author. Please observe the notes on copyright and usage.

Distribution, publication, and copying in any form are prohibited and subject to damages.

© 2024 Ingo Michael Simon
All rights reserved.
Independently published
www.ingosimon.com

Important Notes for Urgent Attention:
The contents of this book are based on the practical experiences of the author with hypnosis applications and psychotherapy in a trance state. Although the author has strived for the utmost care, errors or misunderstandings in the presentation cannot be completely excluded. Therapeutic work with people and the application of hypnosis are solely the responsibility of the hypnotist. It cannot be ruled out that parts of this book may be misunderstood or that the application of a presented procedure may cause an undesirable reaction in the client. The author also assumes no co-responsibility if work with a client is carried out with reference to the statements in this book.

The Author:
Ingo Michael Simon studied psychology and education and is a hypnotherapist with practices in southwestern Germany and Switzerland. With the help of hypnosis-supported psychotherapy, he primarily treats people with persistent psychological conditions. His practice focuses on anxiety disorders, pathological compulsions, and psychosomatic illnesses. His therapeutic offerings mainly include classical and modern hypnosis applications and the dreamland therapy he developed himself.

Copying, publishing, and sharing with third parties are only permitted with the written consent of the author. Please observe the notes on copyright and usage.

Notes on Copyright and Usage

Copying, publishing, and sharing with third parties is prohibited and only permitted with the written consent of the author. Please observe the following copyright and usage guidelines.

This work has been carefully crafted and created to the best of the author's knowledge and personal experience. It comprises text templates and application guidelines for professional hypnosis sessions. The author is a licensed psychotherapist with extensive experience in psychotherapy, coaching, and personal training using hypnotic techniques and methods. Nevertheless, the author and the publisher assume no liability for the accuracy of information, instructions, and advice, nor for any typographical errors. The author and publisher accept no responsibility or liability for the application of these texts and recommendations with clients or patients, nor for any potential consequences or unexpected reactions. It is expressly noted that the application of therapeutic and advisory techniques and formulations lies solely and entirely within the responsibility of the practitioner. This also applies to adherence to the boundaries of legally regulated medical and therapeutic practices. The fact that a book containing action proposals is freely available for sale does not imply that its application with clients or patients is permitted for everyone.

Distribution, publication, and copying in any form are prohibited and subject to damages.

Copying, publishing, and sharing with third parties are only permitted with the written consent of the author. Please observe the notes on copyright and usage.

Distribution, publication, and copying in any form are prohibited and subject to damages.

Table of contents

Introduction 9

#1 11

#2 17

#3 23

#4 28

#5 33

#6 38

#7 43

#8 50

#9 55

#10 60

Overview of All Titles in the Series "Ten Hypnoses" 65

Copying, publishing, and sharing with third parties are only permitted with the written consent of the author. Please observe the notes on copyright and usage.

Distribution, publication, and copying in any form are prohibited and subject to damages.

Copying, publishing, and sharing with third parties are only permitted with the written consent of the author. Please observe the notes on copyright and usage.

Introduction

The series "Ten Hypnoses" is very well known in Germany, Austria, and Switzerland as a collection of texts for therapeutic work and is used by numerous psychotherapeutic practices, doctors, therapists, coaches, and other helping professionals. I am pleased to now be able to offer these texts in other countries as well.

Most therapists have their own methods for inducing and deepening trance as well as for exiting trance. Therefore, I have focused on the main part of the hypnosis. The texts in this book can be integrated as the main part into any hypnosis process.

The texts in this collection use various hypnosis techniques. I will not explain these in detail, as I assume that users have the appropriate training. It is also not necessary to understand the exact structure or functioning of the different parts. The texts can simply be read aloud, and they will have their effect.

Decide for yourself which text best suits your client or patient at any given time. You can also combine passages from different texts. It is not about using all ten hypnoses in sequence. It is a selection of possibilities.

I want to emphasize that books cannot replace therapy. Psychotherapy or other therapeutic treatments involve much more. A careful diagnosis is the necessary basis for deciding on the use of methods, including whether hypnosis or one of my texts should be used. Even in this case, preparatory discussions, follow-up discussions during the session, and of course, a therapeutic concept for the sequence of sessions and the content approaches are essential parts of therapy. This cannot and should not be achieved with a collection of texts.

In any case, I wish you much success in your work and I am pleased if my text templates can contribute in a small way.

Ingo Michael Simon

#1

... ... Today, you want to rest and find new strength ... ... So, first, you concentrate on inner calm and let it become fully conscious ... ... The more you can feel the inner calm, the sooner you will discover new strength ... ... Both are directly connected ... ... You feel calm and find strength ... ... Concentrate once again on the feeling of calm and thus open a door to the new and intense strength deep within you ... ... just like that ... ...

... ... You have decided to finally experience calm and build new strength within it ... ... and it is remarkable how well you are managing to be calm and relaxed right now at this moment ... ... how quickly you have relaxed ... ... how naturally you have gone into trance ... ... and I wonder if you have already noticed how deeply you are in trance ... ... very deep ... ... really very deep ... ... yet you can still hear me well ... ... That is the special thing ... ...

... ... So, you now firmly decide to take care of yourself much more intensively from now on, to notice in time when you need calm again ... ... Just like the feeling at this moment ... ... just calm ... ...

... ... Your thoughts follow your wish ... ... your thoughts focus on sensing your deep inner needs with great attention ... ... including your need for relief ... ... This way, you can react immediately to become calmer, to regenerate sufficiently and intensively ... ... Quite remarkable how well you manage to make this thought a firm ritual already now ... ... a thought that you always carry within you ... ... the thought of taking good care of yourself and taking breaks ... ... In your mind, a plan arises that foresees taking breaks as soon as you feel tired ... ... Right now, you feel tired because you are coming into a deep relaxation ... ... so then ... ... take a break ... ... right now ... ... just like that ... ... right now ... ... just like that ... ...

Now you have time just for yourself ... ... and maybe you have often wondered what to do with time for yourself ... ... how it works to be there for yourself ... ... Now you know how it works ... ... You do the same as now ... ... just rest ... ... that is enough ... ... just rest ... ... that is right ... ... just rest ... ... just like that ... ...

... ... Your body also follows your thoughts ... ... Your body knows this desire for calm and balance ... ... for too long, it has been tired ... ... But the tiredness of your body is positive for you from today, because it shows you that you need to rest now ... ... Truly astonishing how well you can perceive the signals of your body once you pay attention to them ... ... Now you do it ... ... Now you feel your body ... ... You direct all your attention now to your body sensation ... ... and feel your desire for regeneration ... ... your desire for serenity ... ... your desire for calm ... ... your wish for new strength and power ... ...

... ... Your body helps you by sending you clear signals ... ... and it is remarkable how well it can do this and how well it does it ... ... Feel deeply into your body and follow its signals ... ... Pay attention to the signal of tiredness ... ... You can feel it if you now concentrate on this feeling ... ... Your body has already become calm ... ... You no longer move because you are tired and because it is comfortable ... ... So, you feel the tiredness and can make it very intense ... ... The more clearly you feel the tiredness, the faster you can regenerate ... ...

... ... And deep within you, there are many more feelings and sensations for which you now have time ... ... Disappointments ... ... Frustrations ... ... Aggressions ... ... Wounds ... ... Longings ... ... unfulfilled wishes ... ... Whatever is within you, you can feel it ... ... more clearly than ever before ... ... very clearly today, you can feel which feelings arise in you ... ... very old ... ... almost forgotten ... ... but now they are back ... ... also very new ... ... also feelings that are just now arising ... ... at this moment ... ...

... ... You realize that it is important to let all feelings and sensations be there ... ... to allow yourself to feel the way you feel ... ... and to understand all your feelings as friendly messages from your deep inner self, which wants to tell you how you are doing beneath the surface ... ... This helps you finally come to rest ... ... finally recover ... ... Truly astonishing how quickly you manage to simply be ... ... to do nothing, but just to feel ... ... to live in the moment ... ... to regenerate ... ...

... ... Now you are very close to yourself ... ... Your thoughts are clear and relaxed ... ... your body is present and shows you its sensations ... ... Your feelings are the feelings of the moment ... ... You perceive yourself with all your needs clearly ... ... above all, you thus develop a sense of how much calm you need ... ... From this, a plan automatically arises in your thoughts on how you can always find enough calm ... ... through enough breaks ... ... through interruptions ... ... through mindfulness for yourself ... ...

... ... And every morning, when you look in the mirror, you can see it in your own eyes ... ... You can recognize yourself ... ... see your needs and fulfill them ... ... With every glance in the mirror, you connect deeper with yourself and immediately receive a message from your body telling you how it feels ... ... With every glance in the mirror, you connect deeper with yourself and immediately receive a message from your emotions telling you what you feel deep inside ... ... With every glance in the mirror, you connect deeper with yourself and immediately a plan arises in your mind telling you how best to take care of yourself to regenerate ... ...

... ... At any time of the day, you can deliberately look into a mirror to establish a deep connection with yourself, just like now in this moment ... ... and with every glance in a mirror, your mindfulness and sense for yourself grow, so that day by day, you know more clearly and more naturally how you feel ... ... how you design balance and breaks ... ... how you come closer to yourself and your needs for health and satisfaction are fulfilled ... ...

... ... Now once again, direct all your attention to your body and your feelings ... ... Feel and be aware of what you need and how you can act to experience it ... ... You can feel yourself so clearly every day in your life ... ... every single day ... ... just like now ... ... just like this ... ...

#2

... ... The clearer you can imagine this light, the better your subconscious can help you ... ... The stronger you can now build up this image of the universe, the faster you will reach your goal internally as well ... ... because imagination and reality are very close together ... ... very close ... ...

... ... You have decided to build up strength again ... ... This decision is firm ... ... At the same time, you know that you will handle your energy reserves carefully to stay healthy and always be strong ... ... Your decision is good and right because it is true that we can build our own strength ... ... if we know how to do it ... ... Here and today, you can gain strength ... ... firmly anchor strength within you ... ... strength that is simply there and available to you ... ... Remarkable, but it really works ... ... You gain strength from your surroundings ... ... with every breath, you take it in ... ... with every breath ... ...

... ... So, concentrate on your breathing and let it become conscious ... ... feel your breathing with every breath ... ... Inhale ... ... Exhale ... ... [in the client's breathing rhythm, please!] ... ... Inhale ... ... Exhale ... ... Inhale ... ... Exhale ... ... That's good ... ... You are doing it exactly right ... ...

... ... With the next breaths, you take in strength for your mind ... ... Your thoughts become clearer ... ... so clear that you can read them as if on a white sheet ... ... You can perceive and recognize every single thought precisely ... ... even the thoughts you usually had in passing ... ... Now, all thoughts are clear and precise ... ... This way, you feel the increasing strength in your thoughts with every breath ... ... the clarity and purity ... ... the order of your thoughts ... ... Suddenly, everything makes sense ... ... Isn't it nice that you can do this simply by breathing ... ... Inhale ... ... Exhale ... ... and all thoughts become clear ... ... This way, you can recognize which thoughts are only disturbing and sort them out ... ... You simply end all disturbing thoughts and turn to the helpful and constructive ones ... ...

... ... With every single breath, you can feel the strength flowing into you from your surroundings ... ... good! ... ... very good! ... ...

... ... If you think your thoughts should be even clearer and more powerful, then concentrate even more on your breathing and feel the increasing strength ... ...

... ... Now turn to your body ... ... Your body needed rest ... ... Now it can build up strength and energy again ... ... With the next breaths, you feel the strength coming into your body ... ... deep relaxation and strong strength ... ... You feel the calm and relaxation in your body ... ... The more clearly you can feel the relaxation, the faster and better new strength can build up ... ... remarkable that both can happen simultaneously ... ... Feeling calm and building strength ... ... It works ... ... And you are experiencing it right now ... ... Your strength increases with every breath ... ... with every single breath ... ... inhale ... ... exhale ... ... strength and power ... ... just like that ... ... inhale ... ... exhale ... ... Your strength becomes greater and more intense ... ... strength through breathing ... ... strength through breathing ... ... wonderful ... ...

... ... Deep inside you, there is an even greater strength ... ... the strength of your emotions ... ... the greatest energy of our organism ... ... our feelings and sensations ... ... our emotions ... ... You now breathe in and out more deeply than before ... ... even deeper ... ... very deep ... ... just like that ... ... and once again ... ... very deep ... ... This way, strength flows deep into your subconscious ... ... a secret yet active strength that is always available to you ... ... with every breath, you can make it grow ... ... the strength of your feelings ... ... You experience it as a feeling of inner energy ... ... right now ... ... Your energy becomes stronger and stronger ... ... stronger than ever before ... ... right now ... ...

... ... Inhale and exhale ... ... that's already enough ... ... Inhale and exhale ... ... That is already enough ... ... Your organism understands it ... ... excellent ... ... It works exactly as I told you ... ... just inhale and exhale ... ... That is enough ... ... You feel the new strength in you ... ...

... ... You feel how well you can build up strength through targeted breathing ... ... gain new strength ... ... You deeply imprint that this works the same way every day in your life ... ... With a targeted and very intensive breath, you can build up strength and power ... ... with just one breath ... ... deeply in ... ... and out ... ... You try it once again now to get your body used to it ... ... now breathe in deeply ... ... and out ... ... [in the client's breathing rhythm, please, or so that they can follow!] ... ... again, so that your subconscious imprints everything ... ... now breathe in deeply ... ... and out ... ... just like that, and once again ... ... now breathe in deeply ... ... and out ... ... You know how it works ... ... now breathe in deeply ... ... and out ... ... You can do it ... ...

... ... Your deep inner self makes a habit of it for you ... ... This way, you succeed in building strength every day by pausing briefly and breathing consciously ... ... one or maybe two breaths, that's enough ... ... And whenever you breathe in and out deliberately and with the goal of building strength, you immediately feel your inner strength growing ... ... just like now ... ...

... ... Whenever you breathe in and out deliberately and with the goal of building strength, you immediately feel your inner strength growing ... ... just like now ... ...

... ... This way, your strength grows every day ... ... This way, your inner strength becomes more and more natural every day ... ... and you can ensure that it is always built up again ... ... You can maintain and supplement it ... ... every day ... ... You know how simple it is now ... ... just as simple as at this moment, when it works so naturally ... ... You can test it every day … … You can do it again and again … … renew your strength again and again … …

… … Whenever you breathe in and out deliberately and with the goal of building strength, you immediately feel your inner strength growing … … just like now … …

#3

... ... Today, we are working with an anchor, as we have already discussed ... ... You already carry this anchor on your body ... ... your left hand is the anchor that is triggered by the right hand ... ... But we will get to that a bit later ... ... So that you can use the anchor one hundred percent, find the best position now to trigger it ... ... Grasp your left hand with your right hand and feel for the ball of your thumb with your fingers ... ... very lightly ... ... very gently ... ... Decide if you want to grasp the ball of your thumb with your index and middle fingers or with your thumb ... ... maybe you even have another variant ... ... Do it the way you can best grasp your thumb ball ... ... [Wait until the client has found a good grip; prompt again if they do not "participate" immediately] ... ... Wonderful ... ... That works best ... ... very good ... ... And now let go of your hand again and lay both hands loosely next to your body ... ...

... ... Now it is time to find a very deep relaxation ... ... deeper than ever before ... ... You go deeper and deeper into yourself ... ... as if you could sink into yourself ... ... You let go of all thoughts ... ... and imagine how wonderful it will be when you fully succeed in considering yourself important ... ... putting yourself at the center of your care ... ... taking care of yourself completely and enjoying being your best protector ... ... Isn't it remarkable how easily you manage to build this thought? ... ... and just as astonishing is the fact that between a thought and an action, there needs to be only a single second ... ... As soon as you have found a thought or made a decision, you can act ... ... You make it clear to yourself at this moment that you have long made a decision ... ... You have decided to take yourself seriously ... ... to stand up for your health ... ... to take good care of yourself ... ... So, you do not need more than a single second to act on your decision ... ... You immediately do what is necessary to make your decision a reality ... ... to take a break and become calmer ... ... just like now ... ... Now, at this very moment, you can feel that you have already become much calmer inside ... ... Your body lies still, it moves very little ... ... almost not at all ... ... Surely you know that physical movement and inner calm are directly connected ... ... The calmer you are inside, the calmer your body and the slower your movements ... ... just like now ...

… Conversely, it works exactly the same … … If your body slows down because you let it come to rest, your inner feeling also becomes calmer … … just like now … … and the more you concentrate on this relaxation, the deeper it goes … … You have decided to consider yourself important … … that is exactly what you are doing right now, because you are taking this time just for yourself and your relaxation … …

… … It is as if you want to sleep deeply now … … sinking deeper and deeper into the surface on which you lie … … like on a very soft pillow … … like lying on clouds … … sinking deeper and deeper into yourself … … so deep that you perceive my words more and more faintly … … That's good … … Time just for you, because you are important … … Time just for you, because you want to calm down … … Time just for you, because you want to become/ stay healthy … … Time just for you … … just for you … … You feel the deep desire in you to come into this calm and pleasant state faster than now … … How beautiful it can be when you succeed in quickly coming into this wonderful state of relaxation and thus taking care of yourself completely ... ... Truly astonishing that this is actually possible ... ...

... ... You have decided, so you can act ... ... The word 'act' contains the word 'hand' ... ... Now you can actually act ... ... Grab your left hand ... ... Do it now as you practiced ... ... Grasp your left hand and concentrate on your inner feeling ... ... If you think it can become even more pleasant, then just let it become even more beautiful in your feeling ... ... even more relaxed ... ... with even more mindfulness and care for yourself ... ... just like that ... ... just like that ... ... You can do it ... ...

... ... And now let this feeling become fully conscious ... ... and now press the ball of the left hand ... ... and again ... ... press ... ... Your inner self sets itself up so that exactly this pressing of the ball of the hand is the signal to immediately go into the same inner state of calm as now ... ... Whenever you press your hand ball, you immediately go into a state of inner calm and feel the need to treat yourself with mindfulness ... ... to take yourself seriously ... ... to consider yourself important ... ... Your body is relaxed, and your hands are completely calm ... ... Your body has understood how your anchor works ... ... It has already stored it for you, so you can use it again and again ... ...

... ... Whenever you press your hand ball, you immediately go into a state of inner calm and feel the need to treat yourself with mindfulness ... ... to take yourself seriously ... ... to consider yourself important ... ... This will soon become a habit for you, to press or massage your hand ball again and again, it works exactly the same ... ... exactly like now ... ... You have decided ... ... You have acted ...

#4

... ... Today, we are working with an anchor, as we have already discussed ... ... Maybe you are already wondering how quickly this anchor will work ... ... how fast it will be for the scent you will soon learn to help you achieve your goals ... ...

... ... Inner lightness is your goal ... ... You have firmly decided to finally let go ... ... let go of the duties that others can take on too ... ... finally let go ... ... and for you, it is the best decision you could make ... ... It is time to find more free space for yourself and experience your everyday life more calmly ... ... You have long had the desire to work less ... ... to accomplish less ... ... to take on less responsibility ... ... Now it should finally become a reality and remain a reality ... ... Today, you let go ... ...

... ... In fact, you have already started, because you are giving yourself this time just for yourself right now ... ... Attention just for yourself ... ... Freedom just for yourself ... ... So, at this moment, you have let go of your duties ... ... especially the bad conscience often associated with duties because you thought you had to do everything yourself ... ... Today is different ... ... Today is the first day of your new life ... ... a life in which you succeed in

letting go ... ... The good thing is, it is much easier to let go than you thought before ... ... You are experiencing it at this moment ... ... You feel how wonderful it is to let go ... ... just to let yourself drift ... ... and you know that you will find calm with it ... ... calm that enables you to move forward and take on duties when the right time comes ... ... Truly excellent how well you manage to let go of all duties now ... ... to let responsibility rest and simply take a nice break ... ... maybe for a few minutes or for an hour ... ... It can be that simple ... ... And you can let go of even more because now only you are important ... ... Now, you only have one duty ... ... a very special duty that is always there ... ... that is more important than anything else ... ... You have this special duty ... ... You have the duty to take care of your health by letting go ... ... letting go again and again ... ...

... ... Right now, you are setting yourself up to let go of as many duties as possible ... ... But this one remains ... ... It is fixed ... ... the duty to take good care of yourself to stay healthy and to restore health repeatedly ... ... to strengthen it ... ... to secure it ... ... That is the most important duty ... ... And you know exactly how to do it ... ... what you need to do ... ... Let go and take breaks ... ... as often as possible ... ... Let go and take breaks ... ... as often as you can ... ... And it is very often ... ... You make it very clear to yourself ... ... You know it already ... ... You know it must be like this ... ...

... ... Maybe you are wondering how you can calm down and let go immediately in the quickest and best way ... ... Let go of duties ... ... Let go of anger ... ... Let go of resentment ... ... Let go of bitterness ... ... Let go of hurt ... ... Let go of revenge thoughts ... ... Let go of whatever burdens you ... ...

... ... It is easier than you thought ... ... You feel this relaxation now ... ... and if you think it should become even more pleasant ... ... just concentrate even more intensely on this beautiful and pleasant feeling of calm and serenity ... ... Relax even deeper and let go of even more at this moment ...

... ... Feel the calm and the freedom ... ... Letting go brings freedom ... ... Feel this freedom now as intensely as possible ... ... Feel the freedom within you ... ... Breathe deeply and feel your chest expand ... ... This is how good inner freedom feels ... ... This is how good letting go feels ... ... just as free as now ... ... just as free as now ... ... And if you want, it will become even calmer within you, and you will feel how much you have actually let go ... ... You can feel it exactly ... ... You have now let go of all duties and are now taking care of yourself only at this moment ... ... only for yourself ... ...

... ... You can secure it ... ... You can ensure that it also succeeds in your waking everyday life ... ... just like now ... ... every day, just like now ... ... It is very simple ... ... You can go into this feeling of letting go every day and then let go of all thoughts and worries even faster ... ... let go of all duties ... ... let go of whatever burdens you ... ...

... ... [Open the bottle with the aroma and move it towards the client's nose; hold it there] ... ... Now take a deep breath and consciously perceive the scent you notice ... ... a pleasant scent ... ... at the same time, you feel the freedom of letting go in your feeling ... ... Your good feeling and this scent you notice now connect with each other ... ...

They belong together ... ... This scent and the feeling of freedom belong very closely together ... ...

... ... And whenever you smell this scent, you feel calm and freedom deep within you ... ... Whenever you notice this exact scent, you feel the feeling of calm and freedom within you very clearly ... ... Even when you just think of the scent, you can already feel calm and freedom ... ... Your subconscious imprints this scent and connects it with calm and freedom ... ... [Now take the bottle away and close it] ... ...

... ... Continue to breathe calmly and enjoy the calm ... ... Give yourself now mindfulness and attention and trust your subconscious to support you in quickly getting into this state by simply smelling the bottle with the scent I just presented to you ... ... You can even test it ... ... As soon as you perceive the scent, you feel calm ... ... [Open the bottle again and hold it to the client's nose so that they can clearly notice the scent; hold it briefly and then close it again] ... ... That feels good ... ... very, very good ... ...

#5

... ... The clearer you can imagine the sand, the easier it will be for you to take a special step today ... ... a step of liberation and realignment ... ... So, imagine the sand ... ...

... ... You know the difficulties you have had up to today. You also know your goals ... ... You know what you want to achieve ... ... You want to find a good mood again ... ... want to laugh again ... ... want to feel strength and hope again ... ... You want to live ... ...

... ... To do this, it is necessary to change your thoughts and feelings ... ... If you think about it, you understand that your difficulties were mainly the result of disturbing thoughts and feelings ... ... So, you want to let go of these disturbing thoughts and feelings ... ... Maybe you are already curious about how that works ... ... Imagine that each single thought is a small colored ball that is in your head ... ... All feelings are also in your head as small balls ... ... So, you just need to find the disturbing thoughts and feelings to let go of them ... ... You recognize them by their color ... ... Your breathing helps you with this ... ...

… … For example, let's look at your depressed mood … … your tiredness and heaviness … … your inner depression … … So, you can imagine that all the thoughts and feelings that belong to your depressed mood are blue … … In your head, there are many small blue balls that you can let go of … … You breathe in, and the breath flows through your head … … You see it in your mind's eye … … The breath gathers all the blue thoughts and feelings and carries them with it … … And you breathe them out … … They come out of your nose as soap bubbles and float through the room … … Lots of blue soap bubbles … … And one after the other, they pop … … And you continue … … You breathe in and gather all the blue thoughts and feelings … … You breathe them out as soap bubbles … … They float through the room and pop … … You repeat this with every breath. Your depressed mood dissolves more and more … …

… … Your deep inner self is already generating new thoughts … … You feel the feeling of hope … … It happens by itself. You just keep breathing and watching the blue soap bubbles dissolve … … and hope arises … …

… … Now let's look at your feelings of guilt … … because you have often blamed yourself … … maybe you even think now that you have done something wrong or that you are guilty ... ... All thoughts and feelings connected to guilt are yellow ... ... In your head, there are many yellow balls that you can let go of ... ... You breathe in and gather all the yellow thoughts and feelings ... ... And you breathe them out ... ... They come out of your nose as soap bubbles and float through the room ... ... Lots of yellow soap bubbles ... ... And one after the other, they pop ... ... And you continue ... ... You breathe in and gather all the yellow thoughts and feelings ... ... You breathe them out as soap bubbles ... ... They float through the room and pop ... ... You repeat this with every breath ... ...

... ... Your deep inner self is already generating new thoughts. You become free and realize that you are innocent ... ... It happens by itself ... ... You just keep breathing and watching the yellow soap bubbles dissolve ... ... You are innocent ... ... You are innocent ... ...

... ... Next, it's about your perfectionism ... ... You know how it is ... ... You have often tried to fulfill everything particularly well ... ... to do everything better and not to have any omissions ... ... All thoughts and feelings dealing with perfectionism or leading to perfectionism are red ... ...

In your head, there are many red balls that you can let go of … … You breathe in and gather all the red thoughts and feelings … … And you breathe them out … … They come out of your nose as soap bubbles and float through the room … … Lots of red soap bubbles … … And one after the other, they pop … … And you continue … … You breathe in and gather all the red thoughts and feelings … … You breathe them out as soap bubbles … … They float through the room and pop … … You repeat this with every breath … …

… … Your deep inner self is already generating new thoughts. In place of perfectionism comes serenity and consideration for yourself … … It happens by itself … … You just keep breathing and watching the red soap bubbles dissolve … … Serenity and consideration become stronger … … Serenity and consideration become stronger … …

… … Your deep inner self imprints everything … … Deep inside, you know that you can actually breathe out all disturbing thoughts and feelings, today and every day in your life … … You also know that everything you let go of is replaced by new, helpful, constructive thoughts … … Today you can feel it … … So, you can feel it every other day in your life too … … Whenever you want, you simply close your eyes briefly and breathe out all disturbing things as colorful soap bubbles ... ... Just like today, they pop and dissolve ... ... just like today ... ... And you feel new strength ... ...

#6

... ... You can feel this bodily sensation ... ... this sinking ... ... you feel it exactly like that ... ... It shows you how your imagination creates truths ... ... Fantasy and reality are the same ... ...

... ... You are here today to change something. You know the difficulties you have often faced ... ... And you have often wondered how you managed it before ... ... Because there was a time when everything was different ... ... Maybe it was long ago, but you were once balanced and happy ... ... did your work with joy and enjoyed your free time ... ... So, you know that you can change from within ... ... You make it clear to yourself that you already have everything you need for this change ... ... Because there was a time when things were exactly as you want them to be today ... ... So if you could go back to that time to visit yourself and learn from yourself, it could even be easy to awaken this state within you again ... ... You can be the way you were before ... ... First, I will help you go back to that time so that you can experience yourself there ... ... So that you can pick yourself up there ... ...

... ... Imagine you are standing in an endlessly long hallway ... ... In this hallway, there are mirrors hanging on the wall ... ... Each mirror is so tall that you can see yourself entirely in it ... ... You are standing in front of the farthest right mirror and looking into it ... ... You see your reflection ... ... You look at yourself or what you have become ... ... Maybe you don't like what you see or who you see ... ... But that's you ... ... tired and slow ... ... But we will use this slowness today to do everything calmly ... ... in complete calmness ... ... at your pace ... ... in your tempo ... ... Then you slowly walk to the left, step by step, mirror by mirror ... ... Each mirror represents a year ... ... So already in the second mirror, you see yourself a year younger ... ... Then you continue walking ... ... With each mirror, you become a bit younger ... ... Maybe your hairstyle changes more and more ... ... Maybe the color of your hair, and also your facial features slowly become younger ... ... So with each mirror, you go back a year and delve more into your past ... ... Maybe your body changes too ... ... Maybe you were once a bit heavier or thinner ... ... If you go far back, you might even become smaller ... ...

... ... And soon, you will have reached the right time ... ... You see it approaching ... ... That time when you were feeling better ... ... Maybe you are quite a bit younger than today ... ... Maybe you are even smaller because you are a child ... ... Sometimes it is worth going back to a very distant time to find your own strength ... ... So, you arrive at the right mirror and see yourself in it. You recognize yourself, of course ... ... But you look different ... ... You have different feelings, different thoughts, different abilities ... ... This mirror is very special ... ... You can not only look into it ... ... You can step into it and thus enter a world that was very important in your past ... ... So go in ... ... Remember this time ... ... Let it come to life again ... ... Meet yourself and feel that you were once balanced and happy because you respected your limits and knew when you needed a break ... ... when you needed time off ... ... Back then, very different things were important, things that seemed to have been lost over the years ... ... Back then, everything was still in order ... ... and you stand at this point deep within you now ... ... Everything is still in order there ... ... Look at how your younger self thinks, feels, and acts ... ... Even if you see yourself as a child ... ... The child handles your difficulties differently ... ... more naturally ... ... more self-evidently ... ...

... ... You feel all of this within you once again ... ... After all, it is you that you are observing ... ... You make it clear to yourself once more that you are learning from yourself how you can be ... ... How you once were ... ... How you still are deep inside ... ... And how you can always be ... ... You are happy and untroubled ... ...

... ... You stand next to yourself, in a past time that you are reviving here and now, right now ... ... Maybe you already feel this strength ... ... this energy ... ... the magic of change ... ...

... ... You are in your own past ... ... You feel that everything is different here in the past ... ... Everything is better ... ... Just as you want it ... ... But for you, it is the present ... ... Because you are here ... ... You see yourself as a younger person, in the time you are now in ... ... You imagine how this younger person can shape every day of your life ... ... You are this younger person yourself ... ...

You can do all of this ... ... You imprint it on your mind to take it with you on the way back ... ... Then you go back ... ... You pass by the mirrors and can look into them ... ... With each mirror, you become older again and maybe also taller ... ... Your appearance changes ... ... Your hair, your facial features, and also your posture change as you return to the present time ... ... You bring the good and helpful qualities and abilities with you ... ... You can handle all difficulties much better the closer you get to the present ... ...

... ... As you approach the present, make it clear to yourself once more that you can use the abilities you picked up from your younger self every day ... ... Whenever you think you can't go any further ... ... when you feel that your past difficulties could come back again, your subconscious immediately sets out to the time of your greatest abilities and picks you up there ... ...

#7

... ... Make yourself comfortable and place your arms loosely beside your body ... ... Place your palms on the surface and let your hands rest there ... ... [The position of the hands is important for the later ideomotor phase in the main part; the hand position may need to be corrected later, which will not disturb the trance at all. If the client places their hands under the blanket or changes their lying position during the induction and deepening, please ignore it and correct the position only immediately before the planned ideomotor phase, otherwise, you may need to correct multiple times, which would rather produce restlessness. If the client initially took the correct position, they can be easily reminded and quickly find it again later] ... ...

... ... You can observe the ceiling of the room with open eyes and at the same time hear the gentle music in the room. You feel the contact of your body with the surface and can develop a sense of the temperature in the room. At the same time, you go into a pleasant inner calm and relaxation ... ... Now close your eyes and it will become a bit darker, but you can still perceive some of the light through your closed eyes. You can hear my voice clearly and distinctly. As you sink deeper into inner calm, you allow it to become increasingly still within you ... ...

... ... You feel the pillow under your head if you concentrate on it now, and you can also feel the blanket on your body. And you glide deeper and deeper down, letting go of all thoughts and sinking deeper into this beautiful calm state ... ...

... ... You can hear your own breath with each inhalation and exhalation ... ... A part of you relaxes deeper and deeper ... ... with each exhalation, you sink deeper and become calmer and more relaxed ... ... You allow yourself complete calm and relaxation ... ...

... ... It is so simple to enter a pleasant trance ... ... deeper and deeper ... ... Your body knows how to do it and sinks deeper and deeper ... ... so it can become increasingly still within you ... ... calmer and calmer ... ...

... ... If I now say that you should concentrate on your head, you can feel the pillow under your head precisely ... ... Maybe you didn't feel it a minute ago because you weren't paying attention to it ... ... But now you feel it exactly ... ... At the same time, you feel that your head is resting quietly and comfortably ... ... What about your left arm? ... ... Can you feel it? ... ... Of course, you can ... ... Probably, again, you didn't pay particular attention to your left arm a minute ago ... ... But now you can feel it exactly ... ... You know exactly how it feels ... ... Likewise, you can now focus your attention on your right leg ... ... You can feel it precisely ... ... But what about your left arm and what about your head? ... ... You probably notice that you can quickly focus attention on one body part ... ... In doing so, you automatically lose concentration on the other body parts ... ... That is entirely normal ... ... That is also good because we cannot focus on everything at the same time ... ... But you can always do one thing simultaneously ... ... You can go into an increasingly deeper relaxation ... ... precisely because you are directing your attention back and forth, from your head to your arm and your leg, you naturally go into a beautiful deep relaxation ... ... That is the special thing ... ... So now, concentrate on your right arm ... ... and now go on to the left leg ... ... Now you feel your left leg ... ... You can also feel your head again ... ... you just need to direct your attention there ... ... And as you let your gaze and concentration wander back and forth, from your head to your arms, to your legs, or to other body parts, you go deeper and deeper into a wonderful relaxation ... ... This happens simultaneously ... ... That is the special thing ... ...

... ... If relaxation is so easy, how easy is change as well ... ... just as easy ... ... just as easy ... ... Attention, mindfulness, and perception change ... ...

... ... Recently, you have been dealing with yourself and have realized that you should do some things differently in the future ... ... so that you can find the balance between stress and relaxation much better ... ... always taking enough breaks ... ... and feeling immediately when you become weaker and change is essential ... ... You have already succeeded in doing this in your thoughts, and that is really good ... ... Now you can work on developing an inner plan ... ... one that you do not need to think about ... ... Your deep inner self does that for you ... ... Your subconscious can plan anew for you and thereby ensure that you handle yourself and your strength more carefully from the outset ... ... To do this, you need to allow your subconscious to help you ... ... and you have already done that by focusing on your inner calm and your body ... ... So you have already sent a message to your subconscious that it can now work for you in peace ... ... A nice idea that it is not you who is working, but your unconscious side ... ... quietly ... ... You allow it, and precisely because of that, it is also possible ... ...

... ... Now focus your attention on your hands ... ... Check again that they are lying correctly beside your body ... ... loose and comfortable ... ... in complete relaxation ... ... Your palms lightly touch the surface ... ... [If the position was not taken or has been changed, please correct until the hands are loose beside the body.] ... ... Now your subconscious takes the lead ... ... Your deep inner self ensures that old thought and behavior patterns fall away from you and that new ones are built up ... ... without effort ... ... in peace and quiet ... ... Your subconscious ensures that you handle yourself and your inner resources more carefully and makes this new mindfulness and care a matter of course ... ... It is like an inner cleansing ... ... Old patterns of thinking and acting are let go ... ... new patterns of thinking and acting are built up and help you to live freer and happier from now on ... ... balancing and sustainably compensating for stress ... ... working with calm and overview ... ... designing the day more calmly with confidence in inner guidance ... ... Your subconscious now shows you how quickly it progresses in this cleansing and new creation ... ... You will recognize it by the fact that your hands will soon begin to turn outward ... ... Your hands slowly turn outward until they finally lie on their backs ... ... Focus on your hands and just let it happen ... ... Your subconscious begins to turn your hands outward ... ... slowly, at your pace, in your tempo ... ... The more you inwardly adjust to your new thinking and acting, the more your hands turn ... ... They turn more and more outward ... ... Your hands turn with each step of inner change and realignment ... ... exactly so ... ... Feel how your hands slowly turn ... ... They turn outward ... ... as if by themselves ... ... You don't have to do anything ... ... You don't have to undertake anything ... ... You don't have to change anything actively ... ... Your subconscious does everything necessary for you ... ... And as a sign of inner realignment, your hands turn ... ... more and more ... ... further and further ... ... until they lie with the palms facing up ... ... [Observe the turning of the hands, which sets in relatively quickly. The client connects the turning with inner change. Their thinking and feeling adjust to new perspectives, which have already been addressed: balance, calmness, mindfulness! Repeat suggestions about the turning of the hands until they lie on the backs with the palms facing the surface.] ... ... Is it not amazing how quickly your subconscious is willing to help you and even show it to you ... ... So, you can connect with your subconscious ... ... That is exactly what you are doing right now, and your inner self tells you: Yes, I am realigning myself inwardly ... ... Yes, I am taking care of myself ... ... Yes, I give myself mindfulness and care ... ... Yes, from now on, I will take good care of myself ... ... Yes, I will and remain healthy ... ... Yes, I will and remain healthy ... ...

... ... And even in the waking state, you can continue to work on your new strength and confidence by simply consciously turning your hands outward, perceiving them, and reminding yourself that this is a sign of your inner self for change ... ... So, turning your hands can also be a signal for your subconscious to continue working constructively for you and to look after you ... ... Balance, calmness, mindfulness ... ... that is what matters ... ...

#8

... ... You are here today to deal with your old thought patterns and everything that has led to your exhaustion ... ... Everything that is deep in our soul is also found in our body ... ... Every thought, every mood ... ... every single feeling manifests in our body ... ... shows up there as pressure ... ... as tension ... ... as a strange sensation ... ... sometimes as pain ... ... or just as tingling ... ... So if you can clearly feel your body, you can achieve everything ... ...

... ... Somewhere in your body, the old thought patterns of fulfillment also sit ... ... perfectionism ... ... excessive duty fulfillment ... ... extreme care for others and for your tasks ... ... the bad conscience ... ... Let's call it your burnout pattern ... ... It sits deep within you and acts from there without you having noticed it ... ... But now you know it ... ... It is anchored in your feelings and thoughts, but also in your body ... ... You can feel it in your body ... ... Maybe you know that you can feel everything that belongs to you physically, when you come to rest, like now ... ... and focus on your body ... ... like now ... ... Of course, you have experienced how your burnout pattern can affect you in your daily life, but it also shows up in your body ... ... just differently ... ... as tension ... ... as warmth or cold ... ... as pressure or in another way ... ... All thought patterns that we carry deep within us show up most clearly in a specific part of our body ... ... as a signal that we can perceive ... ... So, in your body, a signal of your burnout pattern also shows up, which can warn you ... ... so that you do not burn out again ... ... so that you can take better care of yourself ... ... You just need to recognize this spot, then you can work on it and thus build a new pattern ... ...

... ... Now focus your attention on your body and feel your body ... ... Scan from head to toe, like with a scanner, and find this special spot ... ... Find the spot that feels somehow different because your burnout pattern is there ... ... You will find it ... ... It feels different ... ... maybe just a bit colder or warmer ... ... maybe as a tingling ... ... or as a slight goosebump that suddenly forms ... ... Wherever this spot is ... ... There, your burnout pattern shows up through a physical signal ... ... exactly there ... ...

... ... But even if you haven't found it ... ... It is there ... ... Just take the spot that comes to your mind spontaneously ...

… wherever it is … … Feel deeper and deeper there … … Immerse yourself completely in this feeling … … whatever it may be … … It is your burnout that you feel there … … Immerse yourself deeper and deeper into this spot on your body and feel the signals from your body more and more clearly … … Maybe it feels strenuous or burdensome … … Maybe you thought you had already overcome it more … … Do not worry, because here you mainly feel the thought pattern that led to your overload and exhaustion … …

… … Now focus all your attention and loving care on exactly this spot on your body and connect with the inner pattern that lies there … … Imagine a warm feeling radiating from this spot in all directions … … as if there were an inner sun at exactly this spot, spreading its light and warmth and gently radiating in all directions … … Let it become warmer and warmer, as pleasant as possible … … Imagine bright light radiating from this spot deep into your body … … and also outward … … Let this spot on your body become a source of warmth and feel more and more pleasant for you … … This warmth can encompass your entire body because you bring this mindfulness … … this care for yourself … … So, this spot on your body becomes calmer … … more relaxed ... ... more pleasant ... ... and just as pleasantly, the thought pattern changes ... ... More and more old entanglements dissolve and are replaced by new thought patterns of self-care and mindfulness ... ... Everywhere, where there was the burnout pattern until recently, you find more and more love from you for you ... ... more and more love from you for you ... ... your self-love and mindfulness ... ... your self-love and mindfulness ... ...

... ... You feel the change in your body and make it clear to yourself that your body can always show you how you feel in your emotions ... ... especially in the feelings that you couldn't always feel well in your everyday life ... ... Now you can, because you know that your body helps you ... ... So, every day, you pay attention to your body and ask yourself already in the morning when you get up how your body feels today ... ... It shows you what you need to pay attention to ... ... Whenever you find a spot that feels significantly different from the rest of your body, you give yourself mindfulness and focus on this spot ... ... With that, you connect with the feeling that lies within you and recognize it ... ... So, you can react ... ... So, you can recognize in time when you need to take better care of yourself ... ...

#9

... ... You are preparing for an inner journey ... ... a journey to a faraway land that is simultaneously very close ... ... the land of

your dreams ... ... In the land of dreams, everything is possible ... ... You just need to find it ... ... and you can do that ... ... Feel the rhythm of your breath and follow it ... ... With the wind of your breath, you leave your body and enter the land of dreams ... ...

... ... You stand in a meadow and feel the wind around you ... ... It blows strongly, as if a storm is coming ... ... Maybe it is already a storm, but it doesn't feel like it because you are used to standing in the strongest storm ... ... like a rock in the surf ... ... and naturally, you begin to walk forward ... ... No one has asked you to do so, but you just do it ... ... that is your routine ... ... In your hand, you hold a small burning candle ... ... You carry it with one hand and with the other, you try to protect the flame so that it doesn't go out ... ... It is being whipped by the wind and threatens to extinguish ... ... But you protectively hold your hand over it and continue walking ... ... always further ... ... And you fully concentrate on the candle so that its flame doesn't go out ... ... So often you have felt like a candle in the wind ... ... about to extinguish and always in danger ... ... only your own hands as protection ... ... If you now think about how you have lived and worked in recent years, you can understand it ... ... you can see that you yourself were just like this candle in the wind ... ... exactly like that ... ... But when it was at its worst, you didn't even notice ... ... you were so busy protecting this flame within you that you kept going like a robot ... ... You just kept going, always focused on the candle and always in the wind ... ... There was no time to stop ... ... to rest ... ... to think about yourself and your goals ... ... about what is worth pursuing and what is no longer important ... ... You were like a candle in the wind ... ... about to burn out ... ...

... ... You lift your gaze and look around ... ... You take the risk, even though the wind is so strong ... ... Suddenly, you notice that you are standing in the middle of a forest ... ... You walked into it without noticing because you were focused only on the flame ... ... Now you stop and look deep into the forest ... ... It is dark ... ... You are deep in the land of your dreams ... ... in the forest of your thoughts ... ... but everything is still and dark ... ... as if your thoughts were turned off ... ...

... ... Then you realize that the wind has long since stopped blowing ... ... and you can't even say when it happened ... ... maybe a second ago ... ... maybe a long time ago, who knows ... ... The candle is still burning, and you can look around ... ... look deep into the forest and between the trees ... ...

... ... Between the trees, you see stone tablets, each with an inscription ... ... a word or a sentence ... ... a symbol or a number ... ... They are your thoughts waiting for you here ... ... not the ones you think every day, but the thoughts that have been waiting for you for a long time ... ... for which you have rarely had time ... ... But now you take the time ... ... But because it is so dark here, you take the small candle you are carrying to illuminate these stone tablets and recognize your own thoughts ... ...

... ... Suddenly, you see one thought after another ... ... You can read them individually ... ... and suddenly all the interesting thoughts you once had come back to you ... ...

Ideas ... ... Plans ... ... Wishes ... ... Dreams ... ... You see them suddenly ... ... You feel them suddenly deep within you ... ... as if they are awakening today ... ... With curiosity and interest, you walk between the trees ... ... You leave the path to delve deeper into your thoughts and find new impulses ... ... You use the candle to recognize them all ... ... And suddenly, you realize that the wind is not the real problem ... ... what you need most is time ... ... If you find more thoughts here in the land of dreams, you can only do so as long as the candle burns ... ... But it burns much slower than you thought ... ... So, you have time ... ... and you decide to use your time optimally ... ... for yourself ... ... You know that it is not speed that matters because that would create wind ... ... If you move forward too quickly, the candle could go out and you wouldn't be able to find new thoughts ... ...

... ... So, you firmly decide to handle your time carefully ... ... find peace and balance to wander through the forest of your own thoughts ... ... Maybe you know that thoughts are translated feelings ... ... So, you also find your feelings in the forest of thoughts ... ... feel how you really feel ... ...

… … You wander deeper and deeper into the forest of your thoughts to find more and more thoughts and impulses … … In doing so, you notice that the candle becomes brighter the slower and more carefully you move … … Here in the land of dreams, your candle only burns out if you move quickly … … With calmness and overview … … with interest and curiosity about your thoughts and feelings, it burns eternally … … and with each calm step, it becomes brighter … …

… … Then you consider that this might not only be the case in the land of dreams but also in your everyday life … … Fantasy and reality are much closer together than you thought … … You think about the fact that the land of dreams is deep within you. It has always been there. I am just telling you about it … …

#10

...... You are preparing for an inner journey ...... a journey to a faraway land that is simultaneously very close ...... the land of your dreams ...... In the land of dreams, everything is possible ...... You just need to find it ...... and you can do that ...... Feel the rhythm of your breath and follow it ...... With the wind of your breath, you leave your body and enter the land of dreams ......

...... You are sitting in a glass clock ...... and around you are countless gears that interlock and keep turning and turning ...... endlessly ...... always further ...... You can imagine this clockwork now ...... create a picture in your mind's eye ...... a glass clockwork, and you are right in the middle ...... You can look outside ...... see what is happening around you ...... And yet, you miss a lot ...... The constantly turning and working gears make continuous noises ...... They rattle and clatter ...... They rub against each other ...... They create noise in the drivenness ...... Therefore, you can only see what is outside the glass clockwork ...... you can hardly hear it ...... But maybe you haven't noticed that yet ... ... You think about how it would be to simply stop the clockwork and create calm ... ... The clock would no longer run ... ... Time would stop ... ... You consider whether you might be able to ... ... for a short time ... ... stop the clockwork and take a break ... ... You have probably tried that many times ... ... Just taking a break ... ... or vacation ... ... turning off and doing nothing ... ... finding the right time is not always easy ... ... Then it occurs to you that you might be able to slow down the clockwork ... ... You are in the middle of this glass clockwork and could perhaps just let the gears run slower ... ... Everything would continue ... ... everything with the same precision ... ... just with more calmness ... ... and quieter ... ... so that you could better perceive your surroundings again ... ... and probably yourself too ... ...

... ... And if this clockwork simply ran slower ... ... an hour would still be an hour ... ... just a slow hour ... ... An hour in which you have more time than before ... ... even though everything runs slower ... ... You accomplish the same ... ... and you experience your surroundings actively and feel them very clearly ... ... and you can feel yourself more too ... ... Everything is much quieter when the clockwork runs slower

... ... with the same precision ... ... with the same reliability ... ... and yet an hour remains an hour ... ... and you can accomplish the same within an hour ... ... perhaps even more ... ... in calmness ... ... in complete calmness ... ... Then you might realize that this could be a good idea ... ... And you walk through this huge clockwork and look for a switch ... ... or a lever, with which you can slow down the clockwork ... ... Then you find a golden adjusting screw ... ... It is connected to the tension springs that drive the clockwork ... ... You can tighten them, then everything tightens more, and everything runs faster ... ... You can also loosen them ... ... For this, you have to turn it to the left ... ... then the tension of the springs loosens a bit ... ... Step by step ... ... and everything becomes calmer ... ... The clockwork comes to rest ... ...

... ... Now you turn the adjusting screw to the left ... ... and release the tension ... ... You loosen the tension springs ... ... Everything becomes slower ... ... Everything becomes calmer ... ... The noise decreases ... ... The gears hum very quietly and pleasantly ... ... very calmly ... ... Then you look outside and can see your surroundings ... ... your home ... ... maybe relatives ... ... or friends ... ... There might also be hobbies that interest you ... ... Places and situations ... ... Everything that plays a role in your life, you can see from here ... ... It is, after all, a glass clockwork in which you stand ... ... And now you can look at everything in calmness ... ... And you hear something from outside again ... ... Voices calling you that you couldn't hear before ... ... Maybe you can now also hear your inner voice better, telling you: Take care of yourself! That is what you need most now, and that is what you deserve! ... ...

... ... Then you leave the clockwork and look at your world ... ... Everything is unchanged here ... ... But you have more time because everything runs slower ... ... with the same reliability ... ... and you have gained time ... ... Time for everything that is important to you ... ... maybe for your family ... ... for your friends ... ... for hobbies ... ... for completely new interests and ideas ... ... but above all ... ... for yourself ... ... and that is what matters ... ... You now have time for yourself ... ... Let your clockwork run nice and slowly and comfortably ... ... And maybe it will speed up again at some point ... ... out of routine ... ... because you are used to it ... ... Then you simply come back and go into the glass clockwork ... ... to the golden adjusting screw ... ...

You know now where to find it ... ... And then you slow down the pace ... ... come to rest ... ... very slowly ... ... Just like now ... ... Just like now ... ...

Distribution, publication, and copying in any form are prohibited and subject to damages.

Overview of All Titles in the Series "Ten Hypnoses"

Volume 1: Smoking Cessation
Volume 2: Anxiety and Restlessness
Volume 3: Burnout
Volume 4: Reducing Overweight
Volume 5: Coping with the Past
Volume 6: Suicidal Thoughts and Attempts
Volume 7: Psycho-Oncology
Volume 8: Obsessions and Tics
Volume 9: Self-Confidence and Decision-Making
Volume 10: Grief Work
Volume 11: Psychosomatics
Volume 12: Chronic Pain
Volume 13: Depressive Thoughts
Volume 14: Panic Attacks
Volume 15: Domestic Violence, Victim Support
Volume 16: Post-Traumatic Stress
Volume 17: Exam Anxiety and Stage Fright
Volume 18: Anti-Violence Training, Offender Support
Volume 19: Addiction Tendencies
Volume 20: Social Phobia and Fear of Contact
Volume 21: Nail Biting
Volume 22: Self-Awareness and Self-Love
Volume 23: Teeth Grinding and Night Clenching
Volume 24: Feelings of Guilt
Volume 25: Fear in Crowds
Volume 26: Fear of Flying, Aviophobia
Volume 27: Fear in Enclosed Spaces, Claustrophobia
Volume 28: Tinnitus, Ear Noises
Volume 29: Fear of Heights
Volume 30: Neurodermatitis

Copying, publishing, and sharing with third parties are only permitted with the written consent of the author. Please observe the notes on copyright and usage.

Volume 31: Finding Inner Balance
Volume 32: Overcoming Loneliness
Volume 33: Fear of Illness, Hypochondria
Volume 34: Anticipatory Anxiety, Fear of Fear
Volume 35: Jealousy in Relationships
Volume 36: Driving Anxiety
Volume 37: New Start after Separation
Volume 38: Fear of Injections
Volume 39: Heart Anxiety Neurosis
Volume 40: Overcoming Resentment and Anger
Volume 41: Resolving Blockages and Positive Thinking
Volume 42: Stress Reduction, Stress Management
Volume 43: Body Relaxation
Volume 44: Deep Relaxation
Volume 45: Fear of the Dark
Volume 46: Falling Asleep and Staying Asleep
Volume 47: Compulsive Buying
Volume 48: Restless Legs Syndrome
Volume 49: Bulimia
Volume 50: Anorexia
Volume 51: Overcoming Nightmares
Volume 52: Imagined Deformity
Volume 53: Overcoming Distrust, Finding Trust
Volume 54: Processing Failures
Volume 55: Humiliation, Emotional Hurt
Volume 56: Distressing Compassion, Vicarious Suffering
Volume 57: Self-Forgiveness
Volume 58: Self-Awareness, Self-Confidence
Volume 59: Saying No
Volume 60: Assertiveness
Volume 61: Setting Boundaries and Self-Assertion
Volume 62: Decision-Making Ability

Volume 63: Success Orientation
Volume 64: Ruminating, Circular Thinking
Volume 65: Accepting Pregnancy
Volume 66: Birth Preparation
Volume 67: Spiritual Opening
Volume 68: Joy of Life and Inner Lightness
Volume 69: Patience and Inner Peace
Volume 70: Fibromyalgia and Rheumatism
Volume 71: Irritable Bowel Syndrome, Crohn's Disease
Volume 72: Fear of Nausea, Emetophobia
Volume 73: Stuttering and Cluttering, Speech Flow Disorders
Volume 74: Concentration and Knowledge Anchoring
Volume 75: Vitality and Spontaneity
Volume 76: Searching for Meaning and Finding Goals
Volume 77: Life Crises, Life Events
Volume 78: Workaholism, Goal Obsession
Volume 79: Helper Syndrome, Helpless Helpers
Volume 80: Medication Abuse
Volume 81: Gambling Addiction
Volume 82: Internet Addiction, Smartphone Addiction
Volume 83: Hoarding Disorder, Compulsive Collecting
Volume 84: Conspiracy Thoughts, Overvalued Ideas
Volume 85: Fear of Operations and Treatments
Volume 86: Fear of Aging
Volume 87: Travel Anxiety
Volume 88: Anxiety When Urinating, Paruresis
Volume 89: Fear of Intimacy and Togetherness
Volume 90: Fear of Blushing
Volume 91: Coming Out in Homosexuality
Volume 92: Charisma Training
Volume 93: Migraines and Chronic Headaches
Volume 94: Overcoming Allergies, Bronchial Asthma

Volume 95: Normalizing Blood Pressure
Volume 96: Compulsive Perfectionism
Volume 97: Sports Hypnosis, Motivation
Volume 98: Sports Hypnosis, Performance Enhancement
Volume 99: Determination and Focus
Volume 100: Encountering the Inner Child
Volume 101: Cravings, Binge Eating
Volume 102: Stimulating Metabolism
Volume 103: Bipolar Mood Swings
Volume 104: Borderline, Identity Crises
Volume 105: Hypomania, Euphoria, Mania
Volume 106: Restlessness, Agitation
Volume 107: Nervous Breakdown
Volume 108: Adjustment Disorders
Volume 109: Self-Alienation, Depersonalization
Volume 110: Ending Self-Pity
Volume 111: Primary Gain of Illness
Volume 112: Secondary Gain of Illness
Volume 113: Bullying, Victim Support
Volume 114: Letting Go of Envy and Jealousy
Volume 115: Fear of Spiders, Arachnophobia
Volume 116: Fear of Dogs or Cats
Volume 117: Fear of Strangers, Xenophobia
Volume 118: Excessive Worries, Generalized Anxiety
Volume 119: Strengthening Sense of Responsibility
Volume 120: Unrequited Love, Heartache
Volume 121: Work-Life Balance
Volume 122: Letting Go of Unattainable Goals
Volume 123: Allowing and Accepting Help
Volume 124: Letting Go of Adult Children
Volume 125: Tourette Syndrome
Volume 126: Life Changes and New Starts

Volume 127: Accepting Life in a Wheelchair
Volume 128: Understanding and Overcoming Homesickness
Volume 129: Understanding and Overcoming Wanderlust
Volume 130: Dizziness, Meniere's Disease
Volume 131: Overcoming Aggression
Volume 132: Cutting and Self-Harm
Volume 133: Hair Pulling, Trichotillomania
Volume 134: Postpartum Depression
Volume 135: For Relatives of Dementia Patients
Volume 136: Self-Harm, Artificial Disorders
Volume 137: Activating Self-Healing Powers
Volume 138: Preventing Depression Relapse
Volume 139: Reactive Psychoses, Follow-Up
Volume 140: Obsessive Thoughts and Impulses
Volume 141: Compulsive Checking
Volume 142: Compulsive Counting, Symmetry Obsession
Volume 143: Compulsive Washing, Cleanliness Obsession
Volume 144: Compulsive Questioning
Volume 145: Dissociative Paralysis
Volume 146: Phantom Pain
Volume 147: Overcoming Complaining
Volume 148: Hay Fever, Pollen Allergy
Volume 149: Sexual Abuse, Victim Support
Volume 150: Standing Strong Against Sexism, #metoo
Volume 151: Binge Eating
Volume 152: Overcoming Thoughts of Revenge
Volume 153: Detachment from the Aggressor, Stockholm Syndrome
Volume 154: Courage to Separate
Volume 155: Chronic Fatigue, Exhaustion
Volume 156: Fear of the Future, Existential Anxiety
Volume 157: Excessive Worry About Children
Volume 158: Fear of Failure

Volume 159: Ending Distrust and Control
Volume 160: Dejection, Dysphoria
Volume 161: Boreout, Chronic Boredom
Volume 162: Bipolar Disorders, Relapse Prevention
Volume 163: Mania, Relapse Prevention
Volume 164: Nihilism, Feelings of Worthlessness
Volume 165: Thumb Sucking
Volume 166: Being Brave
Volume 167: Being Proud
Volume 168: Overcoming Shyness
Volume 169: Being Able to Delegate Responsibility
Volume 170: Being Able to Show Emotions
Volume 171: Letting Go of Guilt, Victim Support
Volume 172: Processing Guilt, Offender Support
Volume 173: Mood Swings, Cyclothymia
Volume 174: Lack of Drive, Vital Sadness
Volume 175: Hearing Voices with Reality Reference
Volume 176: Confident Communication
Volume 177: Standing Up for Oneself
Volume 178: Taking New Paths
Volume 179: Confident Job Application
Volume 180: No Longer Being Taken Advantage Of
Volume 181: End of Submissiveness
Volume 182: Depressive Numbness
Volume 183: Mood Drops, Affective Incontinence
Volume 184: Mood Instability
Volume 185: Somatoform Disorders
Volume 186: Stomach Ulcer, Psychosomatic
Volume 187: Accepting Amputation
Volume 188: Overcoming and Letting Go of Hatred
Volume 189: Ending Accusations
Volume 190: Allowing Tears, Being Able to Cry

Volume 191: Finding and Sorting Repressed Feelings
Volume 192: Somatoform Pain
Volume 193: Living Autonomously
Volume 194: Anhedonia, Joylessness
Volume 195: Persistent Sadness
Volume 196: Obesity, Food Addiction
Volume 197: Parents of Abused Children
Volume 198: Letting Go and Letting Be
Volume 199: Childhood Sexual Abuse
Volume 200: Fear of Loss

www.ingramcontent.com/pod-product-compliance
Lightning Source LLC
Chambersburg PA
CBHW030459220526
45464CB00006B/2581